Sometimes
I just stutter

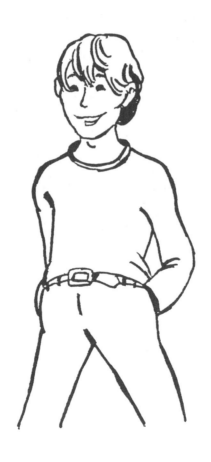

Before you start reading this book...

This book is written for all children who stutter. When you stutter, your mouth doesn't always do what you would like it to do. Sometimes you want to say something and it won't come out. Sometimes you say something and other people make remarks like "Stop stuttering," or "Slow down," or "Just take a deep breath." This usually doesn't help. You often forget what you started out to say. Or you may feel angry or hurt. In the following pages you will find a lot of information about stuttering.

- what makes you stutter
- why sometimes you stutter and sometimes you don't
- why some people have trouble understanding stuttering
- why sometimes you get teased about your stuttering
- that lots of other children stutter too
- that stuttering is sometimes awful and sometimes not

A number of children who stutter have written personal letters for this book. There is lots to learn from what they tell us. I am glad they helped me so much. I have added some information for mothers and fathers, grandmothers and grandfathers, uncles and aunts, brothers and sisters, and also for school teachers. This will help them understand stuttering a little better so they can react in a more helpful way.

You may choose to copy or cut out these pages from the book and address them as letters. Once people have read one of these letters, they may want to read the whole book and learn even more about stuttering.

If you aren't nine years old yet, it may be hard to read all this on your own. In that case, please ask your mom or dad to read it with you.

I hope you will like this book.

Eelco de Geus

Contents

Stuttering is no joke...

Nobody likes to stutter. When you stutter, some words are hard to say. Sometimes it feels like your throat is locked, and you can't get on with what you wanted to say. Or you repeat the first part of a word several times.

When you try really hard to go on talking, you may push through; but more often trying hard just makes things worse. You feel tension in your stomach, and you have to do all kinds of weird things with your mouth or with your whole face to go on talking. Other people can hear that you stutter, and they don't know what to think of it. Often they will try to help you, and sometimes that will be OK. But often it will only make things worse.

People who do not stutter usually find stuttering very hard to understand. They want to help, but they have no idea what they should do. You can see it in their faces—they look puzzled and a bit nervous. When people get nervous they sometimes do dumb things. It's not your fault. It's because they know too little about stuttering. So you should share this book with them. Because when they understand a bit more about stuttering, they will stop getting nervous. And then it is you who will have helped them!

Sometimes you stutter and sometimes you don't...

It is easy to see why people find it hard to understand stuttering. Sometimes you speak quite easily, and at other times talking is difficult. When you play alone in your room and talk out loud, everything is fine. When you talk to a baby or a pet animal, you usually don't have any trouble. When you sing, the words come out fluently. Some children don't stutter when they are angry; for others, being mad will make the stuttering worse. Perhaps it's easy to talk to your younger brother or sister, but you have difficulty talking to grown-ups.

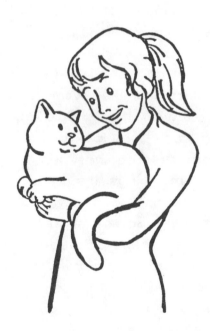

Some children stutter a lot at school and very little at home. Others are fairly fluent at school and stutter most at home. Many children stutter less or not at all during vacation. But many others talk more easily when they go to school every day and stutter more when on vacation. Children who are tired out or sick tend to stutter more, but there are also those who stutter less when they are tired or sick.

Can you take all this in? It is really hard to understand because stuttering comes and goes and seems to be changing all the time. That is why people find it so hard to deal with.

Every child talks in his own way. One speaks slowly, another rapidly. Some children speak in a low voice, others in a loud voice. Everybody has a special way of talking, and every child stutters in his or her own special way. That is just as it should be. Wouldn't it be boring if we were all alike?

What makes you stutter?

All people are different. They do some things well and others not so well. Some children can run very fast; others are not so fast. Some children are good at doing addition or at drawing pictures. Other children find that difficult.

Let's take drawing as an example. To draw well, the muscles of your arm, your hand, and your fingers must work together easily. When you have a hard time drawing a picture, getting all those muscles working together is difficult for you; it is kind of a weak point of yours. It is no big deal—you just need more time to make a good drawing. If you try to do it quickly, there is a bigger chance the picture will not come out well.

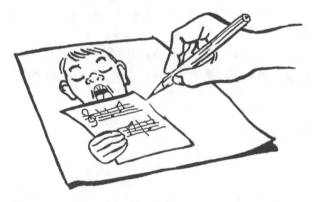

If you are not very good at something and you try to do it quickly, you may get nervous. And when you are nervous things get worse. Especially when you are afraid of making mistakes, you will be more likely to make one. People who are good at drawing do not have these problems. They can draw quickly, even when they feel tense, and they are not at all afraid of making mistakes.

8

It is the same with talking. Some people find it easy—they never have any trouble. But people who stutter have their weak point in the area of speech. It may be difficult at times for your lips and tongue and throat and breathing to work together quickly and smoothly. When you speak slowly or feel at ease, there may be no problem; you may talk just fine. When you talk aloud to yourself, or when you are singing a song, or when you talk to your cat or dog, you feel calm and confident, and you hardly ever stutter.

But when you are in a hurry and want to say something quickly, or when you feel nervous, talking may get harder, and you may start to stutter. And if you are afraid stuttering is wrong and you try hard NOT to stutter, talking will become even more difficult. Then you may shut your eyes, or press hard, or make a face to say what you want. Children who are very afraid of stuttering may avoid talking altogether. They don't pick up the phone, finish their sentences, or they may try to find words that come out more easily. That isn't any fun. So it's much better to just let the stuttering happen and not try to stop it or hide it. You will feel less nervous, and the calmer you are, the easier the talking will be.

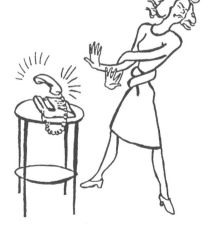

It takes a lot of skill to stutter!

You remember what I said earlier...everybody stutters in a special personal way. Some children say a word or part of a word several times; others block completely. Some children make weird faces; others never do. Some children hate their stuttering so much they would prefer not to talk at all. Others don't seem to mind and just go on talking no matter what.

One might say it takes a lot of skill to stutter.

What is your stuttering like? Look at the following list. There is a circle that can be colored for each stuttering item. You could color the items that go with your own special way of stuttering.

Do you...

- ◯ repeat a sound several times
- ◯ repeat a word several times
- ◯ block on a word
- ◯ puff out some breath before talking
- ◯ shut your eyes when you stutter
- ◯ prolong a sound (s-s-s-s-s-s-ound)
- ◯ move your head around when you stutter
- ◯ move body parts when you stutter
- ◯ stop talking (when you feel stuttering coming)
- ◯ wait for somebody else to say things for you
- ◯ try to find other words

It is quite a feat to stutter, don't you think?
You might try to teach your father or mother to stutter the way you do. You will be surprised how hard it is for them to get it right!

When you feel sad or angry about your stuttering...

People get mad when things go wrong. When you try to do something and you fail again and again, you may be in a very bad temper. People also get to feeling sad inside when things keep going wrong for them.

You would not mind being punished once in a while by your parents or your teacher. But if that happened every day, you would feel upset or angry or both.

Grown-ups usually don't show their anger or their sorrow openly. But if you observe them carefully, you will notice it anyway. They may be more quiet than usual, or they may find fault with everything or want to be alone.

Stuttering every once in a while is no big deal. But if talking gets to be hard very often, you may get mad. Mad at your mouth. Mad at the stuttering. You start to hate it. Perhaps talking gets so hopelessly difficult that it makes you feel sad inside. Sad about your stuttering. People cry when they feel sad. Perhaps you were told not to act like a cry baby but to be brave and strong. But stuttering can feel so bad that it is OK to cry about it. That's nothing to be ashamed of. And it is quite alright to be angry at your stuttering and to hate it. If you express how angry or how sad you are by shouting and stamping your feet or by having a good cry, you will feel a lot better.

Perhaps you don't want other people to know about these feelings. Then why don't you express them in a place where nobody can see or hear you? But it's even better to share your feelings with other people. That will make things easier all around.

Don't be ashamed. Whatever happens, do NOT start blaming yourself. Because it's not your fault that you stutter.

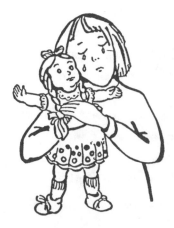

Jenny is seven. She sometimes dislikes her stuttering so much that she gets mad or sad. For her birthday, she got a doll that can move its lips. She calls this doll "Stutterdoll." Every time she feels bad about her stuttering, she goes and tells it all to her doll. If she needs to cry, her doll is there to keep her company. For, of course, it is more comfortable if you don't have to cry alone.

Charles found another solution. He owns a lot of toy cars. When he feels bad about his stuttering, he runs these cars bang crash against each other. Then he pretends the police come to ask what has happened, and he tells them what makes him so mad.

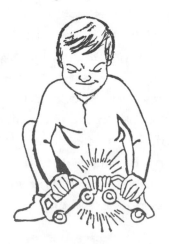

12

When you get teased about your stuttering...

Children tease each other for many different reasons. A child who is taller than the others is sometimes teased. The same may happen to a child who is very short.

You may be teased about a big nose or giant ears. About being sick a lot or about not running fast. About having red hair or about being slow at math. About not wearing the right clothes or about not having a bicycle.

It is pretty normal for children to tease each other sometimes. But if you happen to want a bicycle very much and—on top of that—are teased about not owning one, the teasing really hurts. It is the same with stuttering. When you feel bad about it yourself, it really hurts to be teased about it.

When you are being teased, you can go to the teacher to make it stop, or you can tell your mom and dad and ask them to help you. But you can also do something quite different and tease back. You can always think of something.

I personally think 9-year-old Mark found the best solution. Every time he gets teased he just grins and says, "Come back when you can stutter better than I do." The children stopped teasing him right away!

Some people just don't understand...

You have read that stuttering changes all the time. Every child stutters in his or her own way and even that may change from day to day. People who don't stutter find that hard to understand. People just want things to stay the same. When things keep changing, they get frightened. They do not know how to cope with what they don't understand.

Again, your mom and dad may be worried about your stuttering. They want everything to be OK for you. That is why they, and other grown-ups, and your brothers and sisters, too, often want to help you—partly because they feel sorry for you and partly because stuttering frightens and worries them, and they want it to stop just like you do.

Here are some of the things that people say to help you:

"first take a deep breath"
"take it easy"
"start over again"
"you can do better if you really try"
"stop and slow down"
"now don't stutter like that"
"think about what you want to say before you start"
"now say it over again"

Sometimes it's OK when people say these things. But most often it is not. You are already doing the very best you can. They want you to do even better. Getting on with what you want to say is difficult when you are pushed like that. You might start stuttering even more. Of course these people don't know they are making things harder for you instead of easier. Therefore, it is important to tell them about your stuttering, to explain what you would really like them to do or not do. Then they can be REALLY helpful.

Perhaps it is a bit difficult for you to do this on your own. Just give this book to the people you regularly meet with, or talk it over with your parents. They can inform the other grown-ups around you.

Tim is eleven years old. He stutters a lot more at school than any place else. His teacher did not understand why. Every time Tim wanted to say something in class, the teacher got very nervous and stopped him, and then gave the turn to another child. The teacher thought Tim would be grateful for this because it would save him from having to stutter in front of all the other children.

But it was just the opposite. Tim resented never getting a chance to say something in class. So he talked it over with his mother, and together they went to see the teacher and discussed the problem. They agreed Tim would get a chance to speak any time he wanted to, and that nobody would bother about the stuttering. Tim enjoys going to school now.

It is alright to stutter!

It is not against the law to have big ears. Or red hair. Or blond hair. Or a fat nose. Or expensive clothes and a brand new bike. Or a small nose. Neither is it against the law to stutter. If YOU decide stuttering is wrong, you will put more pressure on yourself not to stutter; and we now know that this will make the stuttering worse. That doesn't make anybody happy. So I always say, "IT'S OK TO STUTTER."

If you decide stuttering is alright, you need not push yourself to talk better. And without that pushing, talking will start getting easier. Just the opposite of what you may have been thinking.

Lydia is ten years old. She was very upset about her stuttering, and she had decided she would not allow it to happen. She was so hard on herself that the stuttering got worse and worse. Her mom and dad agreed with me that stuttering is perfectly alright. We played all kinds of games with stuttering, and recently we made up this poem.

> Just don't splutter,
> Go ahead and stutter;
> Just be bright,
> Stuttering is alright.

We had a good laugh making that up. Lydia is much happier. She does not hate the stuttering as much as she used to, and she speaks more easily already.

You are important!

Because you stutter or because of other things you are not happy with, you may get the idea that you do everything wrong, that you are a wrong kind of person. You think people do not like you. Not only children feel this way. Many grown-ups feel this way too. In that case, you have forgotten something. You have forgotten how important it is that you are alive and that you are you. There is nobody like you in the whole world, you are one of a kind, you are special. You have forgotten that there are many things you are good at and that there are lots of people who love you, like you, care for you.

It's too bad that people often feel too shy to show they care for each other. If you think you do not matter much to anybody and you feel empty inside, remember that you can do something about that. By remembering that you ARE important and if you think so, you will feel strong. If you find it hard to do this on your own, ask your mom or dad, or someone else you trust, to help you remember.

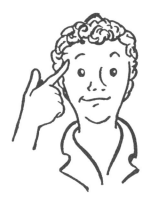

Think of things you like to do and write them down here.

1. _____
2. _____
3. _____
4. _____
5. _____

Think of things you are good at and write them down here.

1. _____
2. _____
3. _____
4. _____
5. _____

And now write down what you think other people like about you.

1. _____
2. _____
3. _____
4. _____
5. _____

Reread a few times what you have put down. You may think of many more things to write. Remember you are important, and remember that people like you because you are you. You are important. DON'T YOU FORGET IT!!!

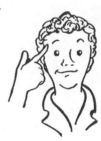

Listen to these kids

I know a lot of children who stutter. Here they tell what they think about stuttering. Perhaps their stories are a bit like your own. Here is what Anne, nine years old, wrote down:

"I don't like to stutter. That is why I want to write about it. Every time I go to see my grandma and granddad, or my uncles and aunts, I stutter when I start to say something. And then I stutter a lot. When I have a fight with kids at school, they call me 'stuttermouth' and I hate that. I don't like stuttering. I think it is embarrassing, and I don't like it. This is the story of Anne."

Sebastian is 13 now. He can explain very clearly what he thinks about stuttering:

"How should I stutter? Some time ago I learned how to stutter more easily and for several years all went well. Now I am older and my stuttering is quite bad again. I have come back for therapy, and I am already making progress. I like the therapy sessions, and that's a good thing, because if you don't like to go, you will probably not profit much from it.

"I would like to get rid of my stuttering. What makes stuttering so hard for me? When I stutter, I usually get stuck. There is a lot of tension in my mouth that keeps growing, and then I am stuck. Stuttering is no joke. But then I say to myself, 'Stuttering isn't against the law, so why shouldn't I stutter a bit?' And that helps.

"Only when I am with people I don't know and they ask me something, do I try very hard not to stutter.

And then I stutter a lot more. When I want to say something very quickly, I get stuck, too. Then people start guessing what I wanted to say. They mean well, but I don't like it at all because I want to say it myself. I used to talk very quickly, but I don't anymore. I have learned to say to myself

> If you don't want to worry,
> Don't talk in a hurry.

"I want to work at my stuttering. I hope to be able to talk more easily someday."

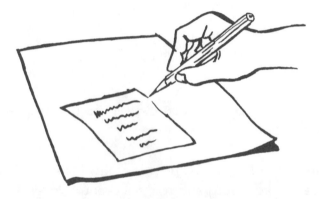

Matthew isn't happy with "all that stuttering." He is 11 now and will go to middle school next year. He comes to see me with another boy. Each week we do all sorts of things together to make talking easier, and we have a good time. Having a good time makes talking easier too. Matthew has written his story here:

"I do not like the stuttering I do, but it won't kill me. I know that now. When I have to read out loud in class I tell myself I won't allow any stuttering. But I stutter anyway and that is what I hate about it. I hope I learn a lot and that it will make me happier. I do not know what more to write, I hope this is enough."

Next comes Eddie's story:

"I'm thirteen years old. I have been stuttering for a long time, about eight years, I think. I started speech therapy when I turned 12. First I went to a lady therapist, but afterwards I went to a male therapist. He keeps telling me it is alright to stutter, but deep inside I think differently. I feel dreadfully ashamed when I stutter. For me it is a real handicap."

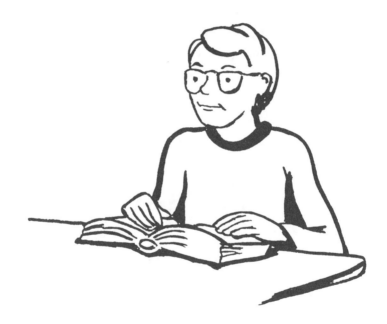

How about your own story...

You have read a number of stories written by other children. But of course you have your own story to tell. It is a good idea to write your own story now. Perhaps you are angry about your stuttering. Then you can write an angry letter. Perhaps you do not mind your stuttering much. You can tell about not minding it. Or perhaps you do not know what to do about your stuttering, or you may want to write down everything you think and feel about your stuttering. That may be a big relief. Just tell your own story, write it down and see what you would like to do with it. You can keep it to yourself or show it to your mom and dad. That's for you to decide.

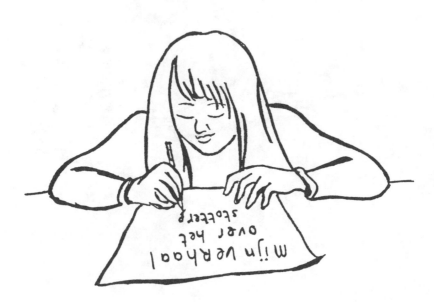

You can also send your letter on to us. We would like you to do that because we learn a lot from reading the stories children who stutter have to tell. And the more we learn from them the better we are able to help others.

Maybe you would like to say something to one of the children who wrote their stories in this book. Just write down what you want to tell or ask them, and send it to us. We will make sure they get your letter. And if you have a lot of questions you can write to us too. Perhaps you are seeing a speech therapist. Of course you can ask them your questions as well. If you do not want to do that, or if you are not having therapy, please write to us. Perhaps we know some of the answers, and then we will write back. You can ask about anything you want. Do you have our address? You can mail your letter to:

Attn: Susie
Stuttering Foundation of America
P. O. Box 11749
Memphis, Tennessee 38111-0749
U.S.A

E-mail: info@stutteringhelp.org
Internet: www.stutteringhelp.org

Who can help you?

It may seem as though you are the only person in the world who stutters. From what you have been reading, you now know that is not true. There are also many people who can help you with your stuttering problem. Of course your mom and dad can help. But sometimes that is not enough. Then you can go to a speech therapist. Many speech therapists know a lot about stuttering and will teach you how to make talking easier for yourself. More importantly, they will listen to what you think and feel about your own stuttering, and they are sure to understand.

They can also help your mom and dad to understand stuttering. And if you have a hard time at school, they can tell the teachers how to make things easier for you. Some speech therapists have specialized in stuttering therapy. (This may give you an idea how complicated stuttering can be!) Anyway, if your stuttering feels like a problem, ask your parents to take you to a speech therapist.

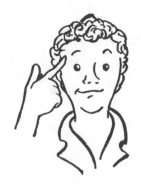

For your brother or sister

Dear Brother or Sister,

I have written this little book for your brother or sister who stutters. Of course you know very well that they stutter. You may have wanted to help when they had trouble talking. What you did or said sometimes made the talking easier and sometimes it did not. Why is that? Your brother or sister has less trouble talking when they feel calm inside. You have probably recognized this. If you have to say something in a large group, you may feel excited or a bit afraid, and it may be hard to find the right words all at once.

You are lucky enough not to stutter in such a situation. Your brother's or sister's speech is more easily disrupted by excitement, worry, or time pressures, and then they often stutter. A lot of things can make you excited or worried...

- An upcoming birthday party.
- School reports that are due.
- The family is about to pack up for vacation.
- Worry / anxiousness about not being good enough at...you name it!
- Feeling sick.
- Being in a hurry.
- Thinking other children don't like you.
- Being afraid of making mistakes.

These are things that can make all of us excited or worried, and then we feel tension inside. But not everybody lets on about these inner tensions. The trouble is that tension always shows up with stuttering. Everybody notices it. And because your brother or sister doesn't want it to be noticed, they will try to stop the stuttering or hide it as best they can. And you know what happens next? They will get more uptight and...the stuttering will get worse. It is quite normal to be excited or worried and uptight. It happens to all of us, to you and to me. But we don't like to admit it. We often think we should naturally be good at everything we do. It stands to reason nobody can be good at EVERYTHING! But all the same, people don't like making mistakes and that makes them uptight when they have to do something difficult.

Because talking is easy for almost everybody, it is hard to believe that some children have serious trouble talking. As soon as there is some tension around, having to talk makes them stutter. You have to do things that make you uptight too, so what's wrong with getting uptight about talking?

If you accept stuttering as something that is perfectly OK with you, your brother or sister will not feel criticized or set apart, the level of tension will drop, and they will not try to hide or stop the stuttering. And that will make talking a lot easier. It is most helpful for them to feel you have some idea of the problem. Thank you for helping in this way.

For fathers and mothers

Dear Father and Mother,

I know you do the best you can to help your child talk more easily. You must be aware of your child's worry and discomfort. Your child will try not to stutter. But the harder he tries, the worse the stuttering is apt to get. This is what makes stuttering such a difficult problem.

It is like wanting to thread a needle. If you are determined to succeed the first time you try, your fingers will get tense, 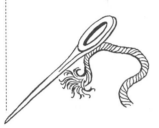 your hand will start to tremble, and of course, this will make it more difficult to get the thread through. You will succeed when you relax and allow yourself to feel calm and self confident, when you allow yourself to be imperfect.

You probably make remarks about your child's stuttering from time to time. It is understandable for you to want to help. Perhaps you don't find it easy to listen to the stuttering and would like it to stop. When you say or do something to help your child, you should observe carefully. If your help results in his becoming more relaxed and calm, you will be doing the right thing. His talking will get easier, too.

It is quite possible your child does not want to be helped when talking. Then it is no use trying to do so. He or she will only get more tense. (Maybe because he gets the message that he is not allowed to be imperfect?) Think of the needle and thread. The more the child tenses up, the harder it will be for the words to come through. Better than any stranger, parents know whether their child is tense or relaxed. That is why we ask for your help. Because you know your child best and can guage his or her feelings, you give the most valuable support of all.

It is important to state that parents' behavior never is the cause of stuttering. Your child was born with a hereditary tendency to stutter. This means the area of speech is a weak point in his general make up. Stuttering manifests itself when demands (in whatever area of life) become too heavy. This stuttering is harmless in itself. But if your child thinks others do not like his stuttering, he will try to talk "better" and to hide or stop the stuttering. That makes the stuttering worse, and it is the reason he still suffers because of it.

So remember you are not the cause of your child's stuttering, but you are the nearest and best supporters on his road to talking more easily. Your child may feel angry as well as hurt and discouraged because of his speech problem. What he needs most are parents who allow him to be resentful or sad about it and who show they understand.

Perhaps your child does not yet have the courage to discuss it with you. But he or she does need to feel your tacit permission to do so. From time to time you may offhandedly ask what he thinks or feels about his stuttering. Make sure the child feels free not to take up the subject if he is not ready to do so. You may be very worried about your child's future. Share your worries with each other and also with a speech therapist. It is important for you as well as for your child not to go on worrying. So try to find competent help soon.

Stuttering manifests itself in so many different shapes and sizes that I can give no more than this general advice. Possibly your child is seldom or never tense, and you may find little of what I have said applicable. But if you feel worried and anxious just the same, do not hesitate to seek the help you and your child are entitled to.

For schoolteachers

Dear Teacher,

You are asked to read this because you have a child in your class who stutters. Stuttering changes from moment to moment and is different in each child. That makes it difficult to deal with. Quite possibly the stuttering of this particular child is no problem for you or for any of the other children. But it is also possible that the other children react to the stuttering and that you yourself are not always sure how best to handle the problem.

Teachers usually have a lot of questions...

> can I be of any help?
> should I make the child read aloud?
> should I talk about the stuttering with the child?
> should I discuss it with the whole class?
> should I ignore the stuttering altogether?
> should I look straight at the child when he stutters or is it better to look away?

These are all legitimate questions. The answers differ for each child who stutters. You could begin by asking if the child has speech therapy, and if so, contact the therapist about what you can or should do. It has often been possible to make a plan by which the child is effectively helped to cope with the school situation.

Most children hate to be set apart, marked as different from the others. So be sure the child who stutters does not get special privileges or is excluded from any class activity. If the stuttering is severe, it is advisable to take the child aside and tackle the issue openly. Some children will appreciate this and feel relieved. Others will refuse to discuss the problem. It's best to respect this and not force the child.

Stuttering is just as hard for the child as it is for you, well, probably harder. So he or she needs all the emotional support they can get. You will help the child by accepting him as he is, and by being warm, understanding and supportive in your attitude towards him or her. You won't have to show this openly, the child will be aware of it and feel more safe. Thank you for your help.

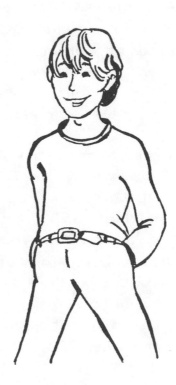

For grandfathers and grandmothers

Dear Grandfather and Grandmother,

Your grandchild needs your understanding and support because he has a serious problem. He has difficulty talking and sometimes stutters a lot. You probably find this hard to understand; most people do. One day your grandchild has hardly any difficulties, another day the stuttering is very prominent and hard to cope with. Please do not think your grandchild can do anything about it. Stuttering is a phenomenon that changes from day to day according to external circumstances, and your grandchild may not have power to modify his speech.

His visit to you may be connected with pleasurable excitement, and any kind of excitement can elicit stuttering. So it is quite possible your grandchild stutters a lot when he is with you. We ask you to understand this, and we hope you will be supportive by not making remarks about the way he expresses himself. If you do, the child will feel pressured to "talk better." That will make him more tense and so increase rather than lessen the severity of the stuttering.

It may be hard for a child to repeat what he has just said because others have not understood it. Stuttering may make your grandchild less easy to understand, especially if your hearing is not what it used to be. Then he may have to repeat the same words several times. Many youngsters find this very embarrassing.

I do not mean to say that you should not ask the child to repeat anything. It is important for you to have real contact. But you can make things easier by paying attention to details like good lighting so you can see each other clearly and have the child right next to you so you can hear better. If the radio or TV is on or the vacuum cleaner going somewhere, you might consider turning them off when you plan to talk together. These details are important in making things pleasant for both of you.

Everything runs more smoothly when we feel relaxed, and this is certainly true for your grandchild's speech. We can relax when we feel safe and at ease. You might consider other means to help your grandchild feel that way when he or she is with you—like giving him a big hug now and again to show your appreciation, by remembering to play his or her favorite game, or by having small outings together. On behalf of your grandchild, I want to thank you for the support you give.

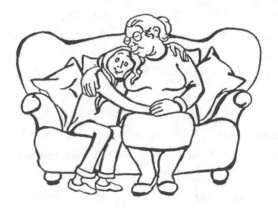

For uncles and aunts

Dear Uncle and Aunt,

Your nephew or niece is bothered by stuttering. You may have wondered about the fact that the stuttering is so variable and very noticeable one day, nothing special the next. You may have observed that the child's speech does not really improve when you try to help by giving advice. This is part of the stuttering problem. We would like to ask you to just accept what happens. Your nephew or niece does not understand what exactly makes the stuttering increase or lessen and doesn't as yet have the power to change their way of talking. We know that it is important to give the child who stutters emotional support. A warm and understanding attitude will do more to lessen stuttering than critical though well-intentioned remarks. It is also important to allow for extra time in the give and take of conversation. The child will feel more at ease, and this will make talking less stressful.

It is alright to talk openly about stuttering when the occasion arises. If no one ever mentions it, the child may get the impression stuttering is so awful it cannot even be discussed. If it is treated like a taboo the child will be convinced it is very bad to stutter. That idea will generate a lot of tension, and thus lead to more stuttering. You can help your nephew or niece by keeping everything around them fairly quiet, by taking ample time when you want to talk together, by choosing a place where others won't rush in unexpectedly, and by keeping eye contact while talking. Of course this is not possible every time you meet, but anything in this direction is helpful.

It will be especially helpful for them to know that you yourself are interested in the problem of stuttering and want to know more about it. They will feel less alone. Thank you for wanting to help.

Fairy tale

Once upon a time there was a boy named Tim,
who lived in a far away country in a large house.
The people he lived with were a sorcerer and a
witch who had stolen him from his parents when
he was a tiny child. Nobody knew about them
because they had disguised themselves as a very
rich and proud couple. To make the disguise more
complete, they had this little boy who had to call
them Father and Mother.

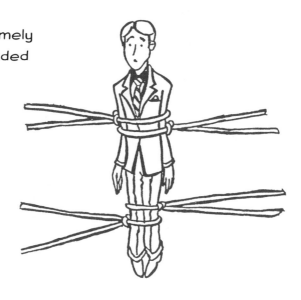

They were extremely
strict and demanded
perfection from
poor Tim. He
was dressed in
the very best
clothes and was
expected to
be polite to
everyone he
met. He had a
brand new bike
but was not
allowed to ride it because it might get dirty.
When people came to the house, they exclaimed
about Tim's beautiful room full of the most exciting
toys. But of course this was all show. Tim was not
really allowed to play with the toys because
something might get broken. And of course, he
could never take other children home with him
because they might damage the expensive
furniture, or his clothes might get out of order.

You will guess he had no friends at school,
and he was often teased by the other kids.
And when visitors came, he was not allowed to
open his mouth because he stuttered. His father
and mother did not want other people to know
their son was not perfect. As you can imagine,
Tim was very unhappy. He thought he did
everything wrong; he was sure nobody liked him.
Sometimes he got angry about it, and sometimes
he felt so lonely and sad that he cried himself to
sleep. He tried very hard to do everything the way his
father and mother wanted, but inside he grew more
and more unhappy.

Then one day a little crooked man came along and
waited for Tim outside the gate of the great house.
He told Tim what we already know—that he had been
stolen by a witch and a sorcerer. He also told Tim
that his real parents had been looking for him ever
since. But lately they had given up all hope of finding
their dear child and had returned home. And then the
old man told Tim that if he had the courage to start
out on his own on a long journey, he would find his
real father and mother who had never stopped loving
him and longing for him.

Tim decided at once to go and find them. He had
had enough of being lonely and unhappy. He grabbed
a suitcase and put his best clothes in it and started
on his way. It was a terribly long journey. He had to
cross dangerous bogs; he had to climb mountains
and wander through wild woods. But every time
he needed food or shelter, he could find what he
wanted as if some invisible person was guiding him.

36

One day he came to a village that he seemed to remember from long, long ago. His heart started beating with sudden hope, and he asked the first person he met if he knew where his parents lived? The young man who answered him stuttered, and when Tim continued on his way he heard other people stuttering too. Soon he was at the door of his old home. What a grand surprise it was to his parents to see their son. That same night they gave a big party in his honor. They had yummy things to eat and everybody was jolly. When he finally got to bed he felt very, very happy.

The next morning he put on his good clothes and was extremely polite to everybody. He sat quietly in a corner and never touched anything because he had been taught not to do so. His mom and dad were surprised and anxious about his behavior. They asked "Why are you so carefully dressed, and why do you sit in a corner? And why don't you go out and play? And why don't you talk with anybody?"

Then Tim told them everything about his life in the big house in that far away country. And his mom and dad said "Now all that is over. You can enjoy yourself and do the things you like to do. And when your clothes get dirty, we don't mind at all, and you can say what you want and talk to everybody. And you do not have to speak carefully, because in this country everybody stutters as much as they please."

Tim was so happy to hear this that he jumped up and down for joy. He rushed out of the house and ran and played and talked as he had never done before. And that night there was another big party because this time Tim truly had come home.
And Tim lived long and happily ever after!

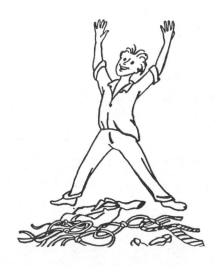

Last message

Stuttering is no joke! So it's important to know you are not alone. There are people who understand you and are willing to help you. It is also important to know that you are not to blame. For your father and mother and all the other people around you, it is important to learn about stuttering. The more they know, the better they will understand what happens, and the better they will be able to help you. Then you will feel certain that it is alright that you are you—whether you stutter or not.

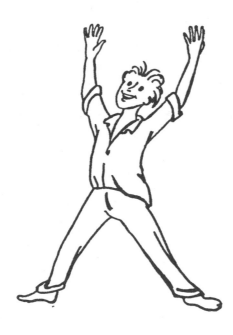

If you believe this book has helped
or you wish to help this worthwhile cause,
please send a donation to

Stuttering Foundation of America
P. O. Box 11749
Memphis, Tennessee 38111-0749

Contributions are tax deductible.

Or donate online at www.stutteringhelp.org

The Stuttering Foundation of America
is a nonprofit charitable organization
dedicated to the
prevention and treatment of stuttering.